HEALTH CARE IN CRISIS:
IS GOVERNMENT THE SOLUTION OR THE PROBLEM?

BY GLENN GRUENHAGEN, CLU, CHFC
Minnesota State Representative

EDITED BY DAVE RACER, MLITT

ALETHOS PRESS
PO Box 600160
St Paul MN 55106

*Health Care in Crisis: Is Government the
Solution or the Problem?*

ISBN 978-0-9702509-6-4

Printed in the U.S.A. by:
Bethany Press International
Bloomington MN

Cover Design and Layout by:
DGRCommunications, Inc.
St Paul MN

http://www.alethospress.com

First Printing

TABLE OF CONTENTS

DEDICATION

This book is dedicated to my children and grandchildren and all young people across this great nation. May this book in some way inspire citizens to persevere in their efforts to bring our state and federal government back to its constitutional limits in order to provide future generations the same opportunities and freedoms that we have been blessed to enjoy.

ACKNOWLEDGEMENTS

I want to thank my wonderful wife, Emily, for her love and tireless prayers, support and critique of my efforts to expose the consequences of the Patient Protection and Affordable Care Act (ObamaCare). To my friend, Daryl Thurn, medical device engineer, for his insights into the venture capital and medical device industry. Finally, to my friend, Dave Racer, for his expertise and insight on the problems and private sector solutions for the U.S. healthcare system. He was truly a blessing during this process.

FOREWORD

A mericans love champions. In sports, it's a first place finish, or at least, a really good try. Fans reward extraordinary talent and a good show. They willingly pay a high price to applaud the best athletes.

In politics, people also search for champions, but, they do not want a good show. They want someone to champion their views and vote in their best interest. Voters want solutions, and predictable, principled politicians. "And keep my taxes low, thank you."

Glenn Gruenhagen is such a champion, and this book gives testimony. In 2010, voters elected him to the Minnesota House of Representatives. They knew him as a family and business man. They knew him as a man with predictable, traditional political values and beliefs.

This book boldly expresses Glenn's principles about U.S. health care. It is informed by his more than 35 years' experience and a mountain of study and reflection.

In this book you will see that Glenn is a man of principle, and unafraid to say so. He is the kind of political champion for which our nation searches every election year.

Dave Racer, MLitt
http://www.daveracer.com

CHAPTER 1
UNITED STATES HEALTH CARE: THE WORLD'S BEST SYSTEM SUFFERS

The United States health care system (if it can even be called that) is like a person – you or me – when we have an upset, sore stomach. No matter how we feel overall, the nagging pain is there, but we don't know what causes it. Do we have a mild case of the flu that will soon pass, or a deadly cancer that will take our life? What we do know is we want it taken care of before it gets worse.

All across the United States, tens of millions of people are receiving high quality health care services every day. Many lives are saved through what sometimes seems like medical miracles. We all know someone who has experienced an incredible change in the quality of their life as the result of modern day health care. So there is much about which we should be grateful. Yet we face serious and significant cost problems in our health care system.

As a nation, we will have spent $2.5 trillion or more on health care in 2011. Health care spending, at 17 percent of our gross domestic product, seems to have no upper limit. We can be sure that

1

total spending will increase in 2012 and every year thereafter, and it is becoming more clear that we cannot afford this.

As a result of the maladies that infect our health care system, an increasing number of individuals and employers are finding it more difficult to afford health insurance. Health care is only one of the multitudes of financial concerns faced by individuals, families, and employers. Yet, it is the unknown nature of human health and the ever-increasing price of care that has left our nation fearful for the future of medical care.

Individuals, families, employers, and government at all levels are struggling to find answers that will retain a high quality and ample quantity of services, but at more affordable prices. Unfortunately, government has chosen to take the lead and, thereby, has created a host of health care reforms that often only make the problem worse. We see this in government run health insurance plans – MinnesotaCare, Medicaid, Medicare, etc. – that too often result in overspending on health care, and driving up the cost for everyone. Or we see government bureaucrats (MediCrats) trying to restrict access to health care services (eventually, denying services) or cutting payments to medical providers in order to save money. The 2010 federal health care reforms passed by Congress, known as ObamaCare, will only make this worse.

Sitting at the center of our current health care finance dilemma are the 78 million baby boomers who began to retire in 2011. As these millions of Americans, who have paid Medicare

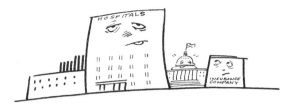

taxes since 1966, began to enroll in Medicare, their health care spending could threaten and cause the collapse of our financial system.

The pain we feel in our stomach is a cancer. We must heal the health care system carefully and properly.

HOW DID WE GET TO THIS PLACE?

The first step in solving any problem is to figure out what created it. Therefore, the first question we must ask is, "How did we get to this place with our health care system?" In other words, to know where we're going we to have to know where we have been.

For nearly 35 years, I have been involved at the grassroots level of health care insurance. My insurance business places me in direct contact with people who consume health care services. As a result, I have watched health insurance premiums spiral upwards, out of control and witnessed the behaviors that drives spending upward.

My practical experience has shown me three critical problems that contribute to the ever-increasing price of health care services and insurance: 1) government funding, 2) government mandates, and 3) government regulation. We cannot move forward to resolve the maladies that plague United States health care system without addressing these three critical issues.

When I started selling health insurance, in 1978, I had the benefit of working with several senior agents. During the 1950s and early 1960s, these agents had sold what are known as individual trust-based health insurance policies, and their primary clients were dairy farmers. Those 1960s health insurance policies paid physicians and hospitals based on a benefit schedule, under "contract law."

Those 1960s insurance policies worked this way: The person paid a premium to the insurance company, and the insurance company paid the physician or hospital when the insured person used medical or hospital services. The insured person, the insurance company, and the medical providers agreed that the insurance plan would pay a flat rate price for each medical service. The insurance contract may have set $5.00 as the price it would pay for an office call. It may have paid $15.00 a day for a hospital stay. Each covered service had a set price like this, and the covered services were known as "usual and customary" – that is, normal medical and hospital services, not experimental or extraordinarily unusual. The individual paid no deductible.

Since those 1960s policies were filed as a trust, the insurance company evaluated health history on a group basis.

INSURANCE: SHORT LESSON #1

The evaluation of health history is called underwriting. Underwriting is an analytical approach the insurance company uses to evaluate risk. The insurance company knows it will spend more to pay for health services for a less healthy individual than for healthy people. Therefore, when the insurance company underwrites an individual case it attempts to segregate less healthy individuals from healthy individuals, thereby limiting the cost of insurance for healthy people. Underwriting, then, protects healthy individuals from severe cost shifting related to paying the cost of care for less healthy individuals.

Those 1960s insurance policies, however, lumped everyone together in a large group, thereby allowing many people with serious health conditions to purchase insurance without any pre-existing condition clause. In other words, less healthy people could purchase insurance through a trust-based group policy at an affordable premium. Sometimes, the insurance company excluded coverage for certain specific medical conditions for an individual.

IMAGINE GETTING ALL YOUR MONEY BACK

The insurance agents' slogan during those days was, "Our company will pay your medical bills, has never had a premium increase, and has never had to change benefits." No one would expect to hear such a slogan today as we have become used to premium increases of five percent, ten percent, or even more every year.

Unlike today, those policies had an incredible feature that seems almost unbelievable today: In addition to paying medical bills, if the insured person kept the policy in force for their entire lifetime, after the insured individual passed away, the company promised to refund the entire premium to the survivors regardless of the total medical claims the individual had incurred. When I first heard this, I could not believe it. How is it possible that an insurance company would never increase your premiums, pay your medical bills, and then refund your entire premium for an individual or family at death? All the senior agents I met confirmed that they had sold this type of insurance policy during the 1950s and early 1960s.

How would you like to own this type of insurance policy today? It cannot, however, happen. The method by which health care is financed changed dramatically as a result of congressional action.

CHAPTER 2
WHAT HAPPENED?

Today, individual and group health "insurance" can cost thousands of dollars a year to cover one person. In some places, a family health insurance plan can cost in excess of $2,000 a month. Nobody expects to gct that money back at the end of their life. Instead, everyone expects the cost to go up every year. There's a reason for this.

Why are we now selling health insurance policies with ever-increasing premiums to cover escalating benefits, with higher deductibles, and no refund of premiums? I asked those senior agents, "When did health care costs start escalating?" They answered unanimously: Congress passed Medicare in 1965, and along with it, Medicaid. In 1966, hospital daily room rates began to escalate, along with the price of every other Medical Service, and they have never stopped going up ever since.

There is a simple, observable fact that drives the cost of health care ever higher. When government programs receive tens of billions of dollars from taxpayers, the individuals and organizations providing the services always increase the price. As payment for health care services shifted from individuals and groups to which they belong, to the government, medical providers raised their prices. This is normal human behavior, but never had to happen. The same fact is observed with other government programs, whether it is for farming, welfare, education, roads and highways, or so-called "economic development;" a list that seems never-ending.

A retired hospital administrator who was active at the time Medicare began explained what he observed. In 1965, Medicare allowed doctors and hospitals to charge a two percent profit for their services. In 1966, however, Medicare eliminated the two percent profit rule from physician and hospital charges as the cost of providing care, experienced by all medical providers, increased. The principle here is well understood: When tax dollars are available to pay for services, there is a temptation to increase charges and fees knowing that the government is picking up the tab. Whether individual physicians, clinics, hospitals or other medical providers consciously act out of greed, or simply see their actions as necessary, the outcome is the same – price inflation beyond all reason. When government spends our tax dollars to benefit a group of people (i.e. medical providers) the physician's personal accountability for his or her spending decisions are transferred to the group. Individual members of the group pressure insurance companies and government to win an increasing share of the pie.

A former hospital board member who served just prior to and immediately after the implementation of Medicare explained the impact of the new law: Prior to Medicare, the local hospital had raised its daily room rate from $11 to $12. This one dollar increase resulted in many of the local expectant mothers choosing to deliver their baby in a neighboring community hospital where the room rate remained at $11 per day. The $1 rate increase eventually led to a loss of patients and revenue. Soon the hospital reduced their room rate back to $11. It is amazing how the free market works when government does not interfere with its corrupting mandates and reimbursements. Unfortunately, Medicare served to eliminate this type of competition. Instead, hospitals began regularly raising their room rates, and why not? Someone else, Medicare, paid the bill, not the patient.

GOVERNMENT PROGRAMS SHIFT COST

When you see a physician, or use hospital services, the provider generates a bill after the fact. When the provider is paid, it's called a reimbursement. Physicians are like anyone else, they want to be paid for their services and not lose money when they see patients.

Unfortunately, when a physician sees a Medicare patient, the government reimbursement is less than is needed to meet their expenses spent to provide the service. Yet, the reimbursement paid to medical providers by Medicaid pays even lower than Medicare.

Here is an example: A family practice physician in Minnesota sees a Medicaid patient, and the government reimburses the doctor $17.00.

If the patient is on Medicare instead of Medicaid, the government reimburses the physician $35.00. However, if the patient has private health insurance the reimbursement will be $54.00. For a person without health insurance, it is common to bill the individual $75.00, or more.

Cost-Shifting: Under our current reimbursement model, the only way a physician or hospital can cover expenses is to charge more for services provided to individuals with private insurance – called cost-shifting. The actual cost of providing Medicare and Medicaid Services is passed on to people with private insurance, and even to a greater extent, uninsured people. (Physicians and hospitals have a hard time collecting from uninsured people, but they have no qualms about charging them the full price.)

One unintended consequence of inadequate reimbursements for Medicare and Medicaid patients is that an increasing number of physicians are refusing to provide services to them. As many as 30 percent of practicing physicians today will take no more Medicare patients, and up to 50 percent refuse to take Medicaid patients. Who can blame them? For every Medicare and Medicaid patient the physician sees, he or she loses income, and runs the risk of not being able to pay the bills. Moreover, the time spent with government subsidized patients eats up time for private pay patients.

Medicare faces a terrible dilemma: Paying for services to as many as 78 million baby boomers, who began retiring in 2011. Congress has known about this problem for many years, and they knew it would create a shortage of doctors. Under ObamaCare, this will become worse.

Current law requires offering Medicaid coverage to individuals earning up to 100 percent of the federal poverty guideline rate. ObamaCare requires states to offer Medicaid coverage to individuals with incomes up to *133 percent* of the federal poverty guidelines beginning in 2014. The Kaiser family foundation projects this will add 22.8 million more people to the Medicaid roles by 2019.[1] National consensus, and numerous reports, indicates that America faces a shortage of 40,000 family practice physicians, or more, by 2020. Medicaid expansion on top of low reimbursement rates is a deadly elixir that threatens access to health care for all Americans.

Physicians and hospitals face the prospect that federal and state governments may, someday, force them to take Medicare and Medicaid patients or risk losing their license to practice. This may seem farfetched today, but it is the type of bureaucratic solution government uses to solve problems.

During 2011, I reviewed the spreadsheets of five hospitals located around my legislative district. Those five hospitals cumulatively lost $63 million providing services to Medicare and Medicaid patients. The hospitals, as much as possible, shifted those costs to private pay patients. This

---

[1] Holahan, J.; Headen. (2010). Medicaid coverage and spending in health reform: national and state by state results for adults at or below 133% FPL." The Henry J Kaiser Family Foundation. Washington, DC. May 2010. P. 13

kind of cost-shifting served to increase private insurance premiums by as much as 40 percent just to offset the losses from Medicare and Medicaid patients.

The president and members of Congress claimed that ObamaCare would cut health care spending $1 trillion during its first 10 years. There are many ways to quibble with that number, but key among them is that the total savings are based on Medicaid reimbursement rates – the lowest rates paid to medical providers. It is easy to see there will be no savings from ObamaCare, only a continuous increase in cost shifting and taxes.

Medicare actuaries have projected that nationwide, 725 hospitals, 2,352 nursing homes and 1,587 home health agencies will become unprofitable and in danger of closing as a result of the Medicaid reimbursement rates in ObamaCare. Just as seriously, polls among doctors project that as many as 40 percent of today's practicing physicians will leave the medical practice if ObamaCare is fully implemented.

ObamaCare will only add to the waste that afflicts our current health care system.

WE TOLERATE IMMENSE WASTE

FACT: PricewaterhouseCoopers recently reported that more than 50 percent of the dollars spent each year in U.S. health care are wasted. In 2010, industry analysts predicted Americans would spend more than $2.5 trillion on health care – half of that is a lot of wasted money.

In December 2004, a Fox News report indicated that physicians and hospitals had overcharged Medicare $20 billion in 2003. I believe the government is aware of this $20 billion boondoggle. Other indications are that Medicare fraud runs to $75 billion or more each year. Instead of reporters using the word "overcharged," they should have called it "ripped off" or "stolen" from Medicare. The Fox News report, remember, dealt only with Medicare, not the scores of other government programs spending millions and billions of additional tax dollars each year. (When Medicaid fraud is added in, the totals lost to fraud are shocking and astronomical.)

Recently, the federal Office of Management and Budget reported on more than 200 federal programs in which 50 cents of every tax dollar spent had been lost to waste and fraud. This extraordinary waste reinforces our Founding Fathers' belief in limited government. As we are finding out, our nation cannot long survive from the fallout of this flirtation with socialism.

There's more: The federal government has basically bankrupted the Social Security Trust Fund. Since 1984, the Social Security Trust Fund collected more in payroll taxes than it paid in benefits, accumulating a $2.5 trillion fund balance. Congress used the Social Security Trust Fund to pay for other government programs. Instead of cash in the bank, the Social Security vault holds I.O.U.s, and these debts must be paid through increased Social Security taxes and from general tax revenue.

It is irrational to believe that the way to fix United States health care system is to give the federal government more money. It is often said that repeating the same behavior that consistently produces the same failed results is a form of insanity.

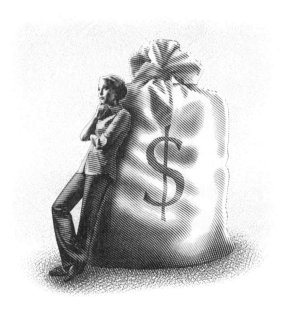

CHAPTER 3
YET WE DID IT AGAIN

On March 23, 2010, a partisan Democratic Congress passed the Patient Protection and Affordable Care Act (PPACA). Incredibly, only a week later, on March 30, Democrats in Congress amended the PPACA. Speaker of the House, Nancy Pelosi, D-California, said, "We have to pass the bill to find out what's in it." I include more about this later in the book.

Would you purchase a health insurance policy where you must pay four years of premiums (taxes) before you could collect any benefits? The overwhelming majority of Americans believe this to be absurd, but that is precisely what ObamaCare asks Americans to do.

The PPACA, known to most Americans as ObamaCare, dramatically raises taxes on everyone during its first four years, before most of its promised "benefits" begin. Congress claimed it would use those four years of increased tax collections to pay the cost of the next six years of benefits. You and I know better: It is foolish to believe that Congress will actually save this money for its intended purpose – remember the social security example. Is it any wonder that the American people hold Congress in such low esteem?

In 1968, Medicare spent $6.2 billion for

health care services for seniors. Its proponents estimated that by 1990, it would spend $10 billion. Instead, Medicare spent $136 billion in 1992 – 1,100 percent more than estimated. In 1968, state and federal governments spent $3.54 billion on Medicaid programs, spending that ballooned to $108.1 billion by 1992 – a 3,050 percent increase in spending.[2]

In contrast to the unbelievable increase in federal and state spending on health care, total Federal spending during the same period, including military spending, increased by only 800 percent.[3]

By 2007, Medicare spent $431.4 billion, and Medicaid spent $326.95 billion.[4] The record of government spending on health care is clear: It will far exceed what its proponents claim. The Democrats in Congress who voted for ObamaCare claimed it would spend an additional $879 billion over 10 years, but this is based on Medicaid reimbursement rates. Medicaid rates are lower than what physicians and hospitals need to cover their costs, and therefore, result in cost-shifting to individuals with private health insurance. History shows us the real number will be astronomical, even unimaginable. As a result, as ObamaCare begins to control health care, federal officials will be forced to ration care. Instead of health care being provided to reduce pain and suffering, and extend

---

[2] Centers for Medicare and Medicaid Services. National Health Expenditures, 1960-2009. Retrieved 10-22-2011.

[3] Retired Minnesota U.S. Senator Rudy Boschwitz provided this information several years ago.

[4] See note 1.

human life, government will be forced to consider a legal concept called "quality of life." ObamaCare will result in the transfer of tens of billions of dollars away from health care and into government bureaucracies. Your care will be based on your age, height, weight, and medical condition. ObamaCare gives authority to set rules regarding the extent of care to a board of 15 unelected bureaucrats called The Independent Payment Advisory Board (some refer to this board as a "death panel"). This board has the power to make health care laws that ration patient options and services.

The rationing that will occur as a result of ObamaCare means that a government bureaucrat, not your physician or you, will make the primary decision about your care based on your age and medical condition. This may mean that medical treatment will be denied. Another way of saying this is that government officials will decide whether tax dollars should be spent on your life. I believe government-run health care should be nicknamed "fat chance" and "good luck."

NOTE: Every government-run, socialized health care system in the world rations medical care. Since 80 percent of lifetime health care expenses occur during the last two years of a patient's lifetime, it is obvious where rationing must begin. As a result, ObamaCare promised to cut $500 billion from Medicare spending. Where will the Washington, D.C. bureaucrats find such a great deal of money without rationing care – to the most vulnerable Americans? In August 2009, *The*

Vancouver Sun reported, "The Vancouver Coastal Health Authority is considering chopping more than 6,000 annual surgeries in an effort to make up for a dramatic budgetary shortfall." Basic logic indicates that 6,000 Vancouver residents will not get critically needed surgeries, at least not right away. They will face long waiting lines, quite common in Canada even for what we consider routine surgeries. Thousands of Canadians each year flee to the United States and elsewhere to get necessary health care.

Lee Kurisko, M.D., wrote an excellent book about the Canadian health care system: *Health Reform: The End of The American Revolution?*[5] In this book, Dr. Kurisko documents the expensive, bureaucratic, government maze that doctors must negotiate to provide necessary health care to patients. Although he is Canadian born and received his medical training there, Kurisko finally left Canada to practice medicine in Minnesota. As he saw the reality of ObamaCare approaching, Kurisko began to question whether the United States could maintain its freedoms while marching toward a Canadian style, government run health care system. We should all be asking that question.

OTHER UNINTENDED CONSEQUENCES

Once Medicare and Medicaid were in place, a host of industries began to flourish. Among

---

[5] Published by Alethos Press LLC, 2009. Available at www.leekurisko.com or www.alethospress.com.

these, the trial lawyers have created immense negative pressure on the health care system. A 2005 survey published in the *Journal of the American Medical Association* indicated that as many as 93 percent of physicians practice defensive medicine. By this, they mean they order tests that may not be necessary, or spend untold hours documenting everything they do, all to avoid a malpractice lawsuit. An August 2008 USA Today article stated that defensive medicine is one of the largest contributors to wasteful spending in our health care system. According to the Pacific research institute, defensive medicine wastes at least $210 billion each year.

The trial lawyers have become one of the most powerful and influential lobbying groups on Capitol Hill, and in each state legislature. Trial lawyers have been successful in most states changing laws that make suing doctors and hospitals a profitable enterprise. Some states, most notably Texas, have begun to limit malpractice settlements much to the chagrin of trial lawyers, but in so doing have managed to hold down some of the increased cost of health care – and attract more doctors.

ObamaCare provided a few million dollars to states to run pilot lawsuit reform programs, but the new law lacks any real litigation reform. Between 1990 and 2010 inclusive, the American Association for Justice (formerly the American Trial Lawyers Association) contributed $33,983,054 to federal election campaigns (this total does not include what attorneys gave as individuals). Remarkably, 89 percent of these contributions went to Democrats.[6] Lawyers ranked the eighth largest group of contributors in the country (and these figures have nothing to do with what is contributed at the state and local level). In contrast, the American Medical Association spent $27,689,135 on campaign donations during the same period, with 53 percent going to Democrats and 47 percent to Republicans.[7] The trial lawyers know where their bread is buttered.

The pharmaceutical companies and medical device industry had many breakthroughs before Medicare/Medicaid. Today, many innovations that could prove helpful in reducing cost or improving health, sit on shelves because no one will take them to market without government approval and Medicare reimbursements. On the other hand, when pharmaceutical companies know that each new patented drug has a reasonably guaranteed market, thanks to Medicare, it provides incentive to create drugs of questionable value.

Today, because a drug or medical device is Medicare approved, people will purchase them even when not necessary. For example, people with sleep apnea find they can receive a "free" CPAP machine. Millions have done so, and it has probably improved health for most of them. Yet, it is common for CPAP supply companies to routinely call CPAP owners to prompt them to spend

[6] Top All-Time Donors, 1989-2012. OpenSecrets.org – Center for Responsive Politics. Retrieved 10-22-2011. http://www.opensecrets.org/orgs/list.php?order=A
[7] Ibid.

more money. The company reasons that since Medicare, Medicaid, or the insurance company covers new masks, headbands, filters, and hoses, the patient should get new ones even while the old ones continue to work. Why not? Someone else pays the cost.

In 1973, Congress passed the HMO Act. By so doing, the federal government extended its reach over health care from Medicare and Medicaid to private insurance. By this, Congress believed it could control runaway spending. How has that worked out? Congress has yet to realize that the main problem is government funding, and the growth of government laws, mandates, and regulations.

During the summer of 2011, *The Wall Street Journal* reported that business and industry spent $1.8 trillion as a result of government regulation. No one, to my knowledge, has reported on how much of the $2.5 trillion spent on health care results from over regulation. One of the outcomes of socialism, however, is an excessive amount of paperwork, and even though technology helps us manage it, it is still very expensive. Between insurance company requirements and government mandates, there seems to be no end to it.

When the first electronic calculators came on the market in the 1960s, they carried a price tag of $200 or more. Today, calculators are available at no cost on your smart phone. If you buy one, chances are you will pay less than $10.00 and it will do far more than an original calculator could ever have done.

Question: What if the government had decided all of those 1960s families had a right to a calculator? If the government had provided a $100 subsidy to every family to purchase one of those $200 calculators do you believe the cost of calculators would have dropped as they did during the next 30 to 40 years, or do you think the price would have gone up?

Government subsidies would have artificially inflated the calculator's price, and kept it from falling. No doubt, calculator costs would have increased even more, creating more demand from people for even greater government subsidies in order to buy more expensive calculators. Milton Friedman, the Nobel Prize winning economist, called this "crony capitalism." It happens when the government chooses economic winners and losers.

Everywhere, we see examples of how technology has reduced the cost of services and products, except for medical technology. Government funding, mandates, and regulations, combined with high malpractice and liability insurance cost, continue to negate the benefits of technology, and drive up its cost in our health care industry.

CHAPTER 4
MUCH NEEDED REFORM

There is an incredible amount of work to be done to fix the U.S. health care system, while maintaining financial security and individual freedom. These are some of the ideas I support:

One: We need to develop a 5 to 10 year plan to greatly reduce or eliminate government funding of the health care industry. We need to reform and reduce government mandates, and reduce the number of laws and regulations imposed on the industry. The goal is to return medical decisions to the physician and patient, rather than empowering insurance companies and government bureaucrats.

We face a funding shortfall of $38 trillion to pay for Medicare's spending from now until 2037. Cong. Paul Ryan, R-Wisconsin, warned Americans that we cannot go on ignoring this pending crisis. He calculates the burden as $335,350 for each U.S. household.[8] More stark is the reality that much of this cost will be borne by young working people. Of those aged 30 and

---

[8] Ryan, P. Roadmap for America's Future. The Budget Committee Republicans. The United States House of representatives. Washington, D.C. January 2011, P 10.

younger today, each carries a burden of $290,000 to pay Medicare's funded cost.

Something has to change. It is immoral to leave this legacy for our new citizens. The truth is that Congress must change the Medicare law.

Gary Burtless, an economist with the left-leaning Brookings Institution, points out, "The Supreme Court has ruled that the U.S.A. does not have a contractual obligation to pay Social Security and Medicare under rules that Congress has no power to change." The Medicare "contract" between the federal government and citizens is real enough, but the terms are variable.

It is self-evident that whichever party controls Congress after the next election will be forced to decide how to solve the Medicare funding problem. The 2010 health care reform law assumes Congress will cut payments to medical providers, but that has not and will not happen. This leaves Medicare administrators with one answer – ration health care to the sickest and most vulnerable senior citizens among us – and that is the wrong solution.

An effective and relatively easy way to reform Medicare is to phase changes in gradually. Let Medicare reduce reimbursements to physicians and hospitals by 20 percent each year for five years. At the same time, allow Medicare recipients to choose Medicare supplemental insurance that will increase its reimbursements by the same 20 percent each year. Medicare patients could have increased choices over deductibles and co-pays, greatly reducing over use, and making better decisions about necessary medical services.

Seniors, just like millions of those under 65 today, should have the ability to buy higher deductible Medicare supplemental policies. They should have access to Health Savings Accounts (HSA).

Some Medicare enrollees may prefer to purchase private health insurance rather than enroll in Medicare. This should be their option, without penalty. For those who choose Medicare, we need to initiate means testing so that wealthy individuals would pay more.

Let doctors charge patients the real price for their services – called balanced billing.

Moving to this system could result in better reimbursement rates for medical providers, and more choices for Medicare patients. Just as importantly, America may have a chance to become financially solvent again one day.

Two: We need immediate malpractice – tort reform. By returning to contract law we could limit medical malpractice liability cost in the medical industry (remarkably, many government agencies are already protected from these malpractice cases). We need to protect patients from dangerous medical practice, and provide help for them when accidents occur. However, trial lawyers should receive a fixed fee for their services rather than contingency fees paid as a percentage of the settlements they win as they sue physicians and hospitals. There should also be financial consequences such as "loser-pays" provisions to discourage individuals from filing frivolous lawsuits.

Three: Health insurance should be portable so that as a person leaves one employer for another they should be able to take their health insurance with them. This is best accomplished by individual insurance policies, instead of employer-provided group insurance. Employers should be enabled to provide pre-tax reimbursement to their employees who then could use these pre-tax dollars to pay for individual health insurance.

We need to gradually move away from employer-provided group health insurance and encourage families and individuals to purchase individual health insurance. They would not lose individual coverage if they change jobs. These individuals will be able to continue health care coverage throughout their working lifetime without having to re-qualify based on their health history.

Four: Individuals should be able to purchase health insurance from any insurance company in the country, across state lines if they choose.

Five: State, not the federal government could provide tax credits or vouchers to low-income people to purchase their own health insurance. These insurance policies could exclude coverage for medical treatment resulting from destructive and unhealthy behaviors – alcoholism and illegal drug use – or the individual could pay a greater premium for this coverage. When an individual enrolls in Medicaid, taxpayers are picking up most of the bill. Medicaid enrollees, then, should be obligated to take random drug tests and lose benefits if they abuse illegal addictive drugs. Medicaid enrollees that refuse to take care of themselves should be required to pay higher co-pays when they visit a physician. Conversely, co-pays should be structured to reward healthy lifestyles.

Six: Minnesota's elected leaders should convince the federal government to allow us to develop pilot programs to privatize federal health care wherever possible, such as providing for nursing home care. This will allow the promotion of innovative alternative ideas and the funding and provision of health care services. For example: When a person needs long-term care, and family members choose to provide it for them at home rather than an expensive facility, those family members should be paid for their services.

Some people today purchase Long-Term Care Insurance. Suppose such coverage pays up to $3,000 a month for nursing home services, but the individual chooses instead to receive care at home from family members. Why not pay a family member $1,000 a month to provide those services? Such a system could greatly reduce the cost of nursing home care.

When an individual qualifies for Medicaid assistance for nursing home care, why not pay a family member to provide that care at home at a reduced rate, rather than at an expensive nursing home? Many families and patients would prefer to do this, but they cannot afford to provide care at home.

It would be possible for professionals to train family members to be stay-at-home medical aides to their loved ones.

Seven: There is a great need to reform the review and approval processes of the Food and Drug Administration. The cost of bringing a new prescription medicine to market approaches $1 billion, and a good deal of that may be driven by inefficient and ineffective testing requirements, paperwork, and other regulatory burdens. The FDA, likewise, drives up the cost of new durable medical devices. We need to ensure that new medicines and devices are safe, and that they serve a valid medical purpose, but the steep price exacted by FDA's bureaucratic process must be reduced.

ALL OF CONGRESS SHOULD GET ON BOARD

Congressman Paul Ryan, R – Wisconsin, is the top Republican on the house budget committee. Ryan introduced his health care reform bill titled "Roadmap for America's Future 2.0." His bill includes some of the above recommendations.

When overhauling the United States health care system it is an overwhelming and daunting challenge. We have no choice. If we do not find better and more affordable ways to deliver health care, our grandchildren will be left living in a second rate society and a lower standard of living.

I expect disagreement about some of what I have written, and expect it to be critiqued, refined, and expanded. The major theme, however, is indisputable: We must get the government out of the health care industry before they totally destroy it.

OBAMACARE CREATES MEDICAL RATIONING

While returning to Minnesota from a 2011 trip to Cleveland, Ohio, I sat next to a cardiac surgeon. He had over 20 years of experience. We discussed ObamaCare and its potential ramifications. The surgeon totally opposed ObamaCare, and said this was true of the majority of surgeons he knew.

As we talked, our discussion focused on the potential for health care rationing as a result of a government-run bureaucracy. The surgeon strongly agreed that ObamaCare would result in rationing of health care to patients. The type of rationing he sees on the horizon will not result from a bureaucrat directly limiting his services, but indirectly, through budget limitations.

The cardiologist suggested how ObamaCare might possibly ration heart surgeries. The doctor said he believes ObamaCare would assign cardiac surgeons in the area to a regional health center. The government would assign a limited amount of expenditures per year for diagnostic tests for cardiac surgeons. Today, the cardiac surgeon orders the tests to make sure surgery is necessary, and to anticipate what kind of surgical procedure to perform. Under ObamaCare, with limits on total dollars to be spent for diagnostic tests, clearly not every patient that meets the test will receive it. It creates two critical situations: Individuals will have to wait for tests and surgery until the funding is in place, and fewer people will receive cardiac surgery.

Consider a year in which ObamaCare bureaucrats only provide enough funding for 50 cardiac diagnostic tests. Yet, the surgeons have 75 patients on their list. Twenty-five of those patients will have to wait until the next year. If during the next year another 75 patients need heart surgery, the backlog will grow to 50. Each year the waiting line grows longer. There is only one winner: funeral service providers.

Whether this is how ObamaCare eventually rations surgeries (and all health services) we cannot know because most of the regulations have not been written yet required to implement ObamaCare. We do know, however, that this is the well-established pattern in Canada and the United Kingdom. Perhaps, however, ObamaCare will simply state that each cardiac surgeon should be limited to a set number of surgeries each year, regardless of the medical needs of people.

When Congress passed ObamaCare, it claimed $500 billion savings from Medicare. Astonishingly, Congress claimed that patients would receive the same or better care than they had previously. This is a complete contradiction in realty and truth. In other words, Congress lied – less money means fewer medical services.

CHAPTER 5:
GOVERNMENT-RUN
HEALTH CARE:
DAMAGING & DESTROYING
TECHNOLOGY & INNOVATION

In 1949, Minnesotan Earl Bakken and his brother-in-law, Palmer Hermundslie, founded a partnership they named Medtronic. They ran their new business out of a garage.

C. Walton Lillihei, M.D., the world renowned cardiac surgeon from the Minnesota School of Medicine urged Bakken to design a battery-powered device to assist heart patients that struggled with irregular heartbeats. In 1960, Bakken patented the pacemaker.

The crude device gave way to incredible innovations in durable medical equipment. Today, Medtronic distributes devices that will stimulate specific areas of the brain, spine, and other organs; shock the heart if it stops; provide blood flow during open heart surgery; scores more and is constantly applying science and technology to devices that improve the health of people all across the world.

Modern medicine depends on applied science developing new devices, medicines, tools, procedures, and understanding of the human body. Just as much, it depends on a free flow of information, also aided by computer technology – the Internet and wireless communications.

Yet, ObamaCare threatens to halt all this, and perhaps, reverse this trend.

WHEN GOVERNMENT OVERREACHES

Author Dave Racer wrote the biography of the Father of the Artificial Heart, Harold D. Kletschka, M.D. (*To Change the Heart of Man* – Kletschka Publishing, 2008). Kletschka, like Bakken and countless other inventors, found the answer to a medical puzzle from an unlikely source – an orange juice machine.

Kletschka noticed how the centrifugal pumping action circulated the orange juice, and set out to design an artificial heart based on the principle. Along with bio-engineer Edson Rafferty, the two men were able to prove their device worked perfectly in animal studies.

Then, in 1975, they faced a dilemma. Congress has passed a new law that placed stringent, difficult, and expensive demands on new medical devices. Knowing that it would take effect in 1976, the two men rushed to get at least the blood pump portion of the heart approved before the new law kicked in. By August of 1975, Texan Denton Cooley, M.D., another world renowned heart surgeon, had used the Bio-Pump® and issued glowing reports. The pump allowed surgeons to stop a person's heart, and yet kept blood flowing during open heart surgery, and it did so without damaging the blood.

Today, ironically, Medtronic owns and distributes the Bio-Pump® and it is the most widely used heart assist blood pump in the world. Unfortunately, Dr. Kletschka died before completing the work on the artificial heart.

Federal government regulation would have driven up the cost of development of the Bio-Pump® from less than $2.5 million to tens of millions of dollars – and far more today. At the very least, its release would have been delayed by years, if not a decade or more.

Yet, ObamaCare threatens these developments with additional regulations and stepped up federal oversight.

SCIENCE, TECHNOLOGY, AND INNOVATION

Technology and innovation are cornerstones of the modern health care industry, and the U.S. economy. Imagine how different our lives would be today if Steve Jobs, Bill Gates, Michael Dell, and so many others had not applied their brains and sheer will to introduce us to affordable, user-friendly computers. Entrepreneurs like these men saw a need, applied their brains to develop hardware and software, and attracted the capital to make it all happen. Their success is a story of our success.

Applied technology increases economic productivity and usually leads to dramatically reducing the cost. Examples abound.

The early Video Cassette Recorders (VCRs) sold for more than $700. Today we purchase Blu-Ray devices for $100-$150 that play high definition movies, and give us direct access to Internet programing. Our cable TV systems provide Digital Video Recording devices (DVRs) for a few dollars a month that can record and store scores of TV programs that we choose.

The evolution of VCRs to Blu-Ray and DVRs illustrates the economic laws of capitalism. American entrepreneurs have duplicated these successes in our economy thousands of times, and we have all benefited.

GOVERNMENT INTERFERENCE

During heavy snows and thunderstorms, people with satellite TV often lose their signals. The storm interferes with the signal in the same manner that government often interferes with the economy. Governments can pervert and distort the laws of capitalism through mandates, regulations, taxes, targeted subsidies, and over-spending.

In our economy, government does have a significant role to play. It must punish those who commit fraud; it must enforce legitimate contracts; it must protect us from domestic violence and foreign invasion; it must ensure equal treatment for our products and service across the world. When government steps in excessively, however, it can damage and even destroy the effects of technology, innovation, and productivity. When this happens, it drives up the cost of services, dampens innovation, and creates unnecessary shortages.

During the summer of 2011, the *Wall Street Journal* reported that government regulations cost our economy $1.8 trillion. This is 14 percent of our Gross Domestic Product (GDP). Two of the most regulated industries are insurance and financial products, and every aspect of health care. How much of our $2.5 trillion in health care spending – 17 percent of GDP – is the result of over-regulation? We do not know, but it is certain to be tens of billions of dollars.

Government over-regulation threatens our health care economy. ObamaCare, however, adds 1,956 new boards and commissions, with estimates of as many as 100,000 pages of new regulations. Perhaps at its root, ObamaCare's purpose is not to improve the U.S. health care system, but to throw it aside and usher in top-down, government-run, bureaucratic health care.

GOVERNMENT CARE IS A POOR MODEL

How and why would U.S. government elected officials want to impose a socialistic government health care plan on the American people? The overwhelming and clear evidence from around the world is that government run health care is ineffective, inefficient, and extremely expensive. Eventually, government-run health care endangers the lives of its most vulnerable citizens by rationing health care treatment.

A November 12, 2011 *Wall Street Journal*

article explains the ultimate futility of government-run health care – and its danger to humans. In *Health System Reflects Greece's Ills*, Charles Forelle explains that the Greek constitution promises free health care for every citizen. Yet, to get that "free" health care, the citizen often must pay bribes to physicians and hospitals. Greece's financial crisis is only adding to the misery, as its government looks to ballooning health care cost as a place to slash spending.

The Greek situation begs the question: When governments run health care, what happens when they run out of money? How much health care money is absorbed by government bureaucracy? How much is wasted in an effort to conform to endless government regulations?

The United States is not Greece, you might say. But ObamaCare sets up the same kinds of federal oversight, implicitly proclaims a human right to health care, and prepares us for the day when the federal government will have to ration health services.

AN EXAMPLE

How would government-run health care damage or destroy medical innovation and limit new technology? Following is a specific example of the creation of a medical device company. Mechanical engineers and medical providers often have innovative ideas of how to treat or improve a medical procedure or device. In this true example, a small number of partners thought they had something unique, and sought funding to develop their new medical idea.

The partners developed a business plan, and took it to the private sector, specifically venture capitalists. Venture capitalists are typically wealthy individuals or groups of investors willing to risk money on startup companies for the possibility of receiving back a high return on their investments. Private venture capitalists provided the partners with $10 million of funding with the requirement that specific goals be reviewed quarterly.

Note that venture capitalists demand results. If these goals and results are not met, all future funding is terminated immediately. Eventually, the venture capitalists invested $40 million in this company. The company needed the money for start-up costs and to help pay the cost of the FDA approval process.

The new company produced three innovative medical therapies to treat cardiovascular diseases. These devices have helped doctors save lives and treat patients more effectively.

As the company grew, it produced 84 new jobs in Minnesota. In 2007, there were more than 100 new start-up medical device companies receiving private venture capital in the Twin Cities Metropolitan area.

Wealthy individuals that are willing to take risks by investing their money in startup companies have created millions of new jobs in a multitude of industries throughout our economy. "Although venture capital represents just 0.02%

of U.S. GDP, it is responsible for an astounding 10% of all U.S. jobs and 18% of U.S. revenues."[9]

Question: When did our country experience almost exponential growth of private wealthy individuals that were willing to invest in startup companies? The answer may surprise you: This began in earnest after President Ronald Reagan pushed Congress to cut taxes on corporate research and development investments along with capital gains tax cuts, and cuts in individual income tax rates. Reagan's efforts led to the greatest economic expansion in U.S. history, which still benefits us today.

The Reagan administration understood the economic and cultural value of the Internet, and approved its use for the private business sector. Until about 1982 Internet use had been restricted to the military. The rest is history.

The Obama administration along with almost all Democrats and a few Republicans propose to increase taxes on wealthy investors – especially on investment income. ObamaCare added a Medicare tax of 3.85 percent on incomes above $200,000 for a single person, and $250,000 for a couple, but this new tax applies to so-called "unearned" income. Unearned income comes from gains related to savings and investment. In other words, ObamaCare takes money from venture capitalists (and others) and gives it to the government. Venture capitalists are smart people, and

---

[9] Grosser, A. (2009) Venture Capital Under Attack. *The Wall Street Journal.* April 16, 2009. Retrieved 11/12/2011.
http://blogs.wsj.com/venturecapital/2009/04/16/guest-column-venture-capital-under-attack/

these new taxes will discourage private venture capital investment.

The Obama team and its Congressional partners would prefer to see the government invest tax dollars and take over the U.S. health care system. This will prove to be a total and complete fiscal and economic disaster for our health care system, but worse than that, it will severely inhibit the development of new technologies as it robs venture capitalists of their earnings. Yes, there will be innovation from individuals working out of their garages, but they will do it with less financial help, and more will fail to ever reach potential.

CHAPTER 6
GOVERNMENT'S WAY

Consider our government-run welfare system. Though it relies on states and local governments to deliver services, they do so under strict regulations and requirements established in Washington, D.C.

In 1965, President Lyndon Johnson declared war on poverty. According to the Heritage Foundation in 2011, the U.S. has spent at least $15.9 trillion on this war since it began. Despite this enormous cost, today's poverty rate is the highest it has been since the 1960s.

Government run welfare programs are like a subsidized surrogacy system that provides financial rewards to women who give birth to children out of wedlock. This creates even more dependency on government. Today, more than 70 percent of births to African-American women are out of wedlock. Dr. Alan Keyes, in *Masters of the Dream*, showed that even during slavery, less than 17 percent of babies were born to single women whose men may not have been married to them (in the sense of civil law) but were with them at birth. In 1965, as the welfare war commenced, Keyes showed that 17 percent of African-American babies were born out of wedlock. Federal welfare programs destroyed the African-American family.

Government welfare programs provide financial support to able-bodied men instead of strong incentives for an honest day's work. Rather than pressure men and women into finding gainful employment, Congress and the president extended unemployment insurance to 99 weeks, providing the incentive to stay home – not go to work. During the summer of 2011, the active workforce in the United States hit an all-time low rate of less than 58 percent of those who could – and should – be working.

Now, through the 2010 Affordable Care Act (ObamaCare) this same inefficient government wants to take over the U.S. health care industry. The results are predictable on two levels: The major problems facing foreign health care systems run by central governments (see Greece, above), and new disincentives to do the right thing for people and for investors. To allow this socialistic philosophy to control our health care system is unwise and un-American.

Venture Capitalists Are Smart People

It is extremely important to understand that private venture capital firms demand some evidence of potential success from individuals seeking money from them: They are risk-takers, but not fools. Furthermore, they demand strong accountability as the business plan unrolls. As government raises taxes on people like venture capitalists, it will destroy their incentive to take risks with startup companies. At the very least, the riskiest businesses with the highest potential rate of return will find doors slammed in their faces.

Imagine if in 1957, Earl Bakken had to deal with today's taxes and regulatory climate, as he tried to convince investors he could stick wires in a person and keep their heart going – moreover, that investors would earn money from it. In today's investment climate, we might still have the hula-hoop, but fewer blood assist heart pumps.

ObamaCare has set us on a course that will seriously damage or destroy the economic engine that creates millions of private sector jobs in the United States.

HOW GOVERNMENT PREFERS TO DO IT

During the late 1980s, Minnesota government agencies spent millions of dollars to build a chopsticks factory in Hibbing, Minnesota. In doing so, they not only wasted tax dollars through direct and indirect subsidies, they obligated Hibbing citizens to pay hundreds of thousands of dollars in mineral taxes over a 50-year period. After a few years, the chopsticks factory closed, but the CEO had made a tidy income during that time.[10] In other words, the State of Minnesota served as the "venture capitalists" for the chopsticks factory, whose investors had very little at stake.

---

[10] Racer, D. (1988) *Poor Rudolph's Alamnack, No. 1: Welcome to Hibbing.* Tiny Press. St. Paul, MN.

In the fall of 2011, we learned that a solar panel company, Solyndra, had gone bankrupt. Our government had used our tax dollars – more than $520 million – to prop up this company. As the story unfolded, we learned of an incredible web of political influence used to make sure that Solyndra got what it wanted. In other words, the United States government served as the "venture capitalists" for this failed company. The outcome was predictable.

Ironically, if Solyndra's founders could have proven to venture capitalists that it had a sound business plan, perhaps it would be on its way to success. We will never know, because the U.S. government violated the rules of the market-place.

Governments tend to make decisions based on political favoritism instead of doing a sober evaluation of risk and reward common to private sector industries.

Government demands very little accountability and simply shrugs its political shoulders when its favored projects fail. As government wastes billions of tax dollars it turns to us and demands more.

REAL LIFE CHOICES ARE PROMOTED

In 2007, there were over 1,000 privately funded venture capital studies in the U.S. currently researching adult stem cells. There is plenty of medical evidence that miracle cures have and will result from these startup companies, and they are doing it in the hope of receiving financial gain.

In contrast, in the area of embryonic stem cell research there are zero privately funded studies in the U.S. Why? Because after more than 35 years of research there is still no medical evidence that medical cures will be developed from embryonic stem cells! Yet, the liberal politicians scream for billions of government tax dollars, most of which will be flushed down the government rat hole of waste, fraud, and abuse.

Chapter 7
ObamaCare's Threat
to Innovation

The new health care law threatens innovation many ways. The "unintended" consequences will not be known for decades. This is just a short list:

1. Taxes levied against durable medical devices drive up their cost.

2. Tens of thousands of pages of new regulations complicate new product development.

3. Income from investments face increased taxes.

4. More experienced physicians, from whom so many new innovations stem, are already leaving the practice of medicine.

5. Younger brilliant innovators will forgo medicine for other fields of study – perhaps in foreign nations.

6. Federal comparative effectiveness studies, and their cold statistical approach to necessary care, ignores individual need and damages the patient-doctor relationship. Government im-

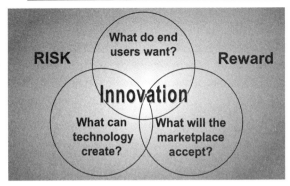

posed rationing, both explicit and implicit, results.

7. The results here in MN have led to substantially reduced venture capital investments in medical device companies.[11]

BRINGING IT HOME

I'd like to give one additional personal example of health care rationing. Recently, my wife visited a doctor to schedule outpatient surgery. I asked the doctor about his thoughts concerning a government-run and funded health care system.

This doctor had immigrated to the United States from Canada. He stated that the Canadian system had limited to no access for patients like my wife who needed surgery. In Canada, he said, my wife would have to wait two and a half years to have her outpatient surgery performed. In the U.S. it had been done in a few months.

[11] Lee, W. (2011) Life Sciences Companies See Financing Dry Up Further. Star-Tribune. Retrieved 11/30/2011. http://www.startribune.com/business/133278438.html

From this experience we receive a strong impression: It sometimes seems that the bureaucrats operating government-run health care hope a person quits seeking care, or in the worst case dies, before receiving the medical treatment.

CONCLUSION: IT'S ON US

As United States' citizens, we have a choice

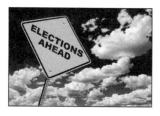

when voting for state and federal elective officials. No matter your personal concerns, certainly this one needs to be in the top three, if not number one: Will the candidate agree to work to reduce government interference in and funding of U.S. health care? Will the candidate commit to doing everything possible to make sure a private health care system, and private health insurance market, can flourish?

If the candidate says "no," then do not vote for him or her. Incumbents that get this wrong should be tossed from office immediately.

Elections have consequences. The decisions we make today will determine not only for ourselves, but also for our children and grandchildren, the type of health care they will receive – and whether we will be able to maintain freedom and liberty for all.

CHAPTER 8:
IS OBAMACARE
A MARXIST
HEALTH CARE SYSTEM?

"From each according to their ability to each according to their need."
Karl Marx, 1875

K arl Marx popularized the idea that society owns a person's production, property, and income and, therefore, has a right to redistribute it to others. Marx's idea aligns with the present-day liberal dogma that governments should tax the "rich" – productive labor – to give to others, even if they are able-bodied and nonproductive.

Marx's idea directly contradicts The Declaration of Independence that asserts we are endowed by our Creator with the unalienable right to the pursuit of happiness. By this, the Founding Fathers made direct reference to the individual right to earn from his or her labor, and own the production of that labor. The Drafters of the Constitution incorporated this idea into the Bill of Rights, which provides specific protections for private property – the Fourteenth Amendment further solidified this idea.

49

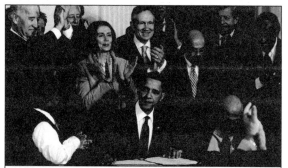

President Barack Obama signs the Patient Protection and Affordable Care Act of 2010 surrounded by politicians and representatives of special interest groups. Since then, many of its flaws have been exposed.

Marxism, then, relies on a principle that stands completely opposed to our form of government, our traditions, and that which has made us a strong nation: The right to own our own production.

Congress passed the Patient Protection and Affordable Care Act on March 23, 2010, and amended it a week later. The original bill ran to more than 2,700 pages. Its number of pages is only an emblem of its real destructive nature. It is in the thousands of words where threats to our freedom and property lie.

ObamaCare (the name adopted by nearly every faction to describe the 2010 law) must stand up to Supreme Court scrutiny. Yet, it has already produced untold negative effects atop those indicated in the previous two chapters. By the end of 2011, the federal government will have expended tens of billions of our tax dollars to implement its provisions. The Obama Administration rushes to put them into place, knowing that it is nearly impossible to repeal programs once established.

ObamaCare, as a federal program, will magnify itself exponentially compared to attempts by states to reform their own health care programs. As such, it is also an attack on the rights of citizens to rely on local governments – towns, cities, counties, states – to deliver health care services. Instead, ObamaCare attempts to force a one-size-fits-all plan across the country. It has already started to crumble, but its threats to freedom are quite real.

DIGGING INTO OBAMACARE

Following is a partial list of provisions that Congress passed in 2010. In addition, other references are made to the new powers granted to the federal Secretary of Health and Human Services – the title is mentioned more than 3,000 times in the new law, making it the National Heath Care Czar.

1. A 15-member unelected board will set the parameters of national health care services and financing. Section 1889A established the Independent Payment Advisory Board, appointed by the President, and empowers it to make medical coverage decisions for Medicare and Medicaid. These decisions always bleed out into private health care.

2. Decisions about how physicians and hospitals will deliver care are made subject

to "comparative effectiveness information" – Section 399HH. This means that a federal agency will decide what type and how much care is appropriate, and provide physicians and hospitals with federally-approved guidelines on how to administer it.

This idea has its roots in the British National Health Service, a system known for its stinginess toward providing care to those with serious medical conditions. The British National Institute for Comparative Effectiveness (NICE) is the government agency charged with deciding whether individuals whose health conditions are deemed too expensive to justify the system spending additional health care dollars on treatment. NICE, thereby, makes life and death decisions for British citizens.

The PPACA's comparative effective testing is sure to result in withholding treatment – rationing – as government bureaucrats decide how much care is cost efficient. These decisions are based on the individual's age, weight, and health condition.

For the overwhelming number of Americans, approximately 80 percent of their lifetime health care costs are incurred during the last few years of their life – often as much as 60 percent during the last few months of life. As government bureaucrats decide the appropriateness of the use of health care dollars, the result will be rationing health care to patients during the final weeks, months or years of their life. This is a subtle form of euthanasia.

Former New York Lieutenant Governor, Betsy McCaughey, M.D., spotted Congress intent in an early version of the bill. She found a provision on page 425 of the proposed health care bill that everyone on Social Security (including all Seniors and SSI recipients) would be required to go to MANDATORY counseling every five years for the purpose of choosing ways to end suffering – and life. McGaughey's revelation sent a warning shot across Congress bow. Congress eliminated the specific provision, but laid the groundwork to incorporate some of the outcomes in a provision that could result in federal wellness requirements for Medicare enrollees.

3.   Section 4202 sets in motion a federal takeover of health and wellness programs for individuals deemed at risk. It provides federal grants – taxpayer's money – to evaluate the health of individuals in two distinct groups: aged 55-64, and those on Medicare. Individuals are also directed into programs that the federal government determines will improve their health outcomes. Those without insurance are enrolled in public plans, or ushered into private health insurance if they can afford it – most will purchase taxpayer-subsidized coverage.

It is in programs like this that truly, the devil is in the details. The Secretary is required to report to Congress no later than September 30, 2013 on the results of a number of demonstration projects. The recommendation contains language that should chill any rational freedom lover: The secretary will make "… recommendations for such legislation and administrative action as the Secretary determines appropriate to promote healthy lifestyles and chronic disease self-management for Medicare beneficiaries."[12] This sets in motion the potential for the Secretary to create requirements for each individual relative to how they must live if they wish to continue receiving Medicare and other federal benefits.

4.   Congress and the President claimed the PPACA would spend only an additional $879 billion over its first 10 years (based on Medicaid reimbursement rates). Detractors widely ridiculed this claim from the beginning of the debate. To reach this number, Congress said it would cut $500 billion by reducing payments to physicians and hospitals. Congress perpetrated this hoax knowing that already, nearly 30 percent of physicians refused to see new Medicare patients because of the low reimbursements they were receiving. Within months of passing the PPACA, Congress restored a good chunk of those proposed "savings" when it allowed increased reimbursements to take effect.

Of the $500 billion Congress claimed

---

[12] PPACA. Section 4202(b)(3), Consolidated Print version, p 470.

PPACA savings would produce, only one percent is projected to come from eliminating waste, fraud, and abuse! Yet, estimates of Medicare and Medicaid abuse range from $75 billion to $175 billion annually. This is the track record of government funded health care. No matter what government does, in almost every case it is five to ten times more expensive than if produced or delivered through the private sector. The private health care industry needs to make a profit to stay in business and, therefore, has a greater incentive to eliminate waste, fraud, and abuse, unlike the government.

5.   The PPACA establishes 1,968 new boards, agencies, and study groups. New government bureaucracies include: The National Health care Workforce Commission, The Medical Advisory Council, The Interagency Coordinating Working Group on Health care Quality, Patient Safety Research Center, Shared Decision Making Resource Center, and the Center for Health Outcomes Research and Evaluation -- (see diagram at the end of this chapter). The new health care bureaucracy will require hiring tens of thousands of new government union employees paid from tax dollars and increased health care cost. This new funding feeds the unions with millions in dues, and provides liberal politicians with a ready stash of campaign dollars. The PPACA is a sure source of support for liberal politicians whose primary goal is to be reelected, not to provide citi-

zens with effective, efficient and lifesaving medical treatment.

6. The PPACA promises better health outcomes as a result of science. Health science requires mountains of medical data, each collected from individuals that use health care facilities. The PPACA claims to protect individual medical records, and perhaps it will at the outset. There is no guarantee that over time, your private health information will be protected from the scrutiny of government bureaucrats who will use it to make decisions about you – about your health care. Evaluating private health care data can lead to unprecedented government control over individual lives.

7. If the health care services you need are outside government guidelines one of the new federal boards may deem them fraudulent. Your physician could possibly be fined or barred from practice for recommending treatment outside the proposed government guidelines. Imagine the restraints on medical practitioners whose treatments fall outside of the norm set by the American Medical Association or other powerful physician lobbies – chiropractors, naturopathic doctors, and the like. Much of what passes as a medically approved treatment will be subject to endless political lobbying by powerful interest groups whose members' livelihood depends on winning bureaucratic approval.

8.   More than 11 million Americans have Health Savings Accounts (HSA) today. These have provided a great incentive to spend health care dollars wisely. The PPACA threatens HSAs, especially for low- to middle-income individuals that will receive tax-subsided health insurance. This has to do with complicated technical issues related to several sections of the new law. Suffice it to say, millions of Americans will be denied the choice of an HSA because of the PPACA.

9.   In Subtitle D, "Available Coverage Choices for All Americans," the PPACA establishes a vast new, hugely expensive insurance distribution system. The health insurance exchanges envisioned by the new law are said to be flexible, and highly influenced by each state so that there will be 50 unique organizations distributing health insurance. In reality, each exchange must be approved by the Secretary, and as such, must comply with a labyrinth of regulations.

The exchanges exist for a single purpose – to use taxpayer dollars to buy down the cost of insurance premiums. Once hooked on government subsidies, no one wants to give them up, and will never support a candidate who promises to eliminate benefits, no matter how unaffordable they have become.

Liberals in Congress believed that exchanges would help millions of uninsured afford coverage, but ignores reality. Unin-

sured individuals fall into many categories –
one sticks out: These are people that do not
want to spend money on insurance. Why
would they be expected to purchase subsidized insurance? Even $10 a month is more
than they spend today, and many will face
premiums of hundreds of dollars a month.

For those that do take advantage of subsidized health insurance premiums, they will
forever be subject to it. No one will willingly choose to disqualify themselves from a
government handout such as this.

Exchanges make it more convenient for the
federal government to micro-manage health
care and insurance companies. Congress
claims exchanges create competition among
insurance plans, but requires stringent rules
about Qualified Health Plans, resulting in
cookie-cutter insurance and few incentives
for real competition.

Subsidizing exchange health plans requires
taxing private insurance companies. In other
words, premiums must go up to include the
new taxes, making insurance more expensive, not less.

In "government speak" exchange-based insurance is said to create "equal competition." The federal government makes the
rules, takes your money, uses it to fund its
bureaucrats, gives the balance to someone
else, and then manipulates the system into
what they want it to do. This is Marxism,

not the freedom and liberty to which we've grown accustomed.

10. The PPACA raises taxes in numerous ways. It creates additional taxes on medical devices, health insurance policies, and prescription medicines. Some view these new taxes as justifiable since big corporations pay them, but that is a myth. All of these taxes are passed along to health care consumers as increased prices for medical devices, increased insurance premiums, and costlier prescription medicines. Individuals pay all of these taxes, not the corporations which only serve to collect them.

Section 9105 of the PPACA directly increased the tax burden of individuals and couples. Individuals earning more than $200,000 a year and couples earning more than $250,000 will see their payroll tax increase by .9 percent (above the income thresholds). But there is more. It also increased their payroll tax rate by an additional 1.45 percent on individuals and their employers (2.9 percent) on income above the thresholds. Many of these earn their incomes from small businesses and so, pay both the employer and employee share of the taxes, meaning a total increase of 3.85 percent tax on income above the thresholds. But there is more.

The Medicare tax applies only to wages and salaries, except for these "high income" individuals (above $200,000 and $250,000 respectively). The new tax will apply to all income above the thresholds, no matter how it is earned. This means income from dividends, savings, investments, real estate, and such, are all subject to the additional 3.85 percent.

What about average-income earners that sell a house or other property and have a gain greater than $250,000 (for couples). It appears they, too, will be subject to the additional 3.85 percent on all income above the threshold. Grandma and Grandpa, selling their lifetime home, could find themselves saddled with a one-time tax payment as a result (at least, only on the portion that nets them $250,000 or more in income).

Taxes transfer productive money in the private economy to money spent by government bureaucrats. This will especially hurt small business that creates the majority of jobs, robbed of investment income for new jobs and equipment. The PPACA also imposes new mandates and fines on business related to providing health care. The result of all this new taxation will be reduced hiring and layoffs for small and mid-size business. More of our jobs will go overseas.

11. The federal Congressional Budget Office (CBO) strongly disagreed with the Democratic Congressional majority about the projected 10-year cost of ObamaCare. Congress, of course, claimed the CBO had projected only $879 billion in additional

spending. In projecting the cost at $879 billion, the CBO simply adopted the assumptions dictated to it by Congressional Democrats. In computer programming, this is called "Garbage In, Garbage Out." Subsequently, the CBO applied more realistic assumptions and found the increased cost to be at least $1.5 trillion. Republicans insisted the real increase in spending amounted to at least $2.5 trillion. We cannot know but based on the projections of government in terms of costs for other past programs, the CBO's projection is probably far too low.

12. The Obama administration owes Planned Parenthood for its election successes. Therefore, it had hoped to mandate coverage of abortions under the PPACA, using your tax dollars to kill innocent unborn children. As a compromise, President Obama issued an Executive Order that purports to ban abortion funding under the PPACA. Pro-lifers see this as a slight of hand, and expect pro-abortion advocates to push for federal funding of abortion.

13. The PPACA creates mega-medical provider structures called Accountable Care Organizations (ACOs). The ACO forces physicians into huge corporate medical structures and imposes strict guidelines on them. The ACO's primary objective is to provide efficient health care services, meaning spending less to get more results. Already, experienced physicians are indicating they plan to retire or enter a cash, or non-in-

surance medical practice. The ACO movement is well underway, as corporate medicine spends billions getting ready for full implementation of ObamaCare. Higher paid physicians are finding they have no place in the newly formed ACOs, operating on their federally-posed strict budgets. Doctors will be rewarded financially for rationing health care (gatekeepers). Doctors who don't support rationing will be penalized.

"Nationwide physician shortages are expected to balloon to 62,900 doctors in five years and 91,500 by 2020, according to new Assn. of American Medical Colleges work force projections."[13] Projections vary, with consistent reports of a lack of 45,000 family practice physicians alone by 2020. These statistics are fairly easy to validate, since the physicians that would fill these positions are not in medical school today, and it takes 14 years on average to train a physician.

Atop the previously reported shortages stands the stark reality that the PPACA attempts to enroll 32 million uninsured individuals into subsidized health plans. The current shortage, then, is made worse when millions more seek "free" preventive health care offered by the PPACA.

Fewer physicians leads to health care rationing or downgrading of quality as medi-

---

[13] Krupa, C. (2010) Physician shortage projected to soar to more than 91,000 in a decade. Amednews.com. The American Medical Association. Washington, D.C. Retrieved on 11/26/2011. http://www.ama-assn.org/amednews/2010/10/11/prsb1011.htm

cine turns to professionals with less training than received by physicians.

14. The CBO report issued at the end of 2008 related to health care reform served as Congress' bible. Page xv of that report stated that to save money, the services of professional health insurance agents would probably be eliminated. This assumes that the insurance agent does nothing worthwhile for their clients, but sucks money out of the system. Ask anyone with private health insurance if that is true. Then ask them how they will enjoy dialing a federal government office to get help in dealing with insurance companies, physicians, hospitals, pharmacies, and all the other work agents do for them today. For every private insurance agent eliminated, 25 to 30 government union employees will need to be hired to replace them.

15. The Employee Benefit Research Institute found that public employees receive benefits that cost 230 percent more than those paid by private employers. In other words, a private employer can provide benefits to 2.3 employees for every one government employee. Government employees receive their pay from tax dollars. We cannot afford tens of thousands of new bureaucrats required by the PPACA.

16. A study done by the Coalition for Health care Redesign (COHR) indicates that health insurance exchanges will discriminate

against married couples. *The Wall Street Journal* (January 2010) reports that married couples could pay as much as $10,000 more in annual insurance premiums compared to unmarried couples. The exchange health plans, then, encourage co-habitation, and discourage traditional marriage similar to other federal welfare programs.[14]

17. ObamaCare seeks to grant the Secretary of Health and Human Services tremendous discretionary authority to regulate health care workers. Forced unionization, along with compulsory union dues, may quickly become a required standard forcing hundreds of thousands of physicians and nurses across the country to join unions.

18. Perhaps it sounds trivial and to some, a good idea, but when you think about it, Section 4205 should send shivers down your spine. In this section, the PPACA gives the federal Secretary of Health and Human Services unprecedented power to regulate what you eat, at least at national chain restaurants. This micro-management of huge segment of the private economy allows the secretary to set menu items and regulate their recipes.

The intention of Section 4205 is to reduce obesity. In fact, much of the PPACA focuses on governments finding ways to influence

---

[14] Racer, D. (2011) Health Insurance Exchanges. Facts tell us to re-think potential outcomes. The Coalition for Healthcare Redesign. St. Paul, MN. 7/1/2011. P 3.

(force, persuade, cajole, penalize) individuals to live healthier. We all could use a good dose of healthy living, but do we really want an appointed federal official – the Secretary – to tell us what we can eat? Such is the PPACA, intruding on many individual choices and freedoms, all in some insane sense that the government knows better how we should live than we do ourselves.

19. The PPACA calls for increased taxes at several levels. The Internal Revenue Service collects those taxes. It also requires individuals to purchase health insurance, and expects to use taxpayer funds to subsidize coverage for more than 30 million people. It expands Medicaid by adding eligibility for individuals earning up to 133 percent of the Federal Poverty Guideline. Since subsidies and Medicaid are related to individual income, the PPACA had to provide billions of dollars so the IRS could hire as many as 15,000 new employees to ensure compliance with the new law.

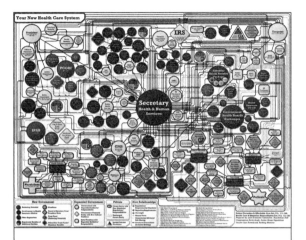

This chart, prepared by the Congressional Joint Economic Committee, shows the complex new government bureaucracies created by the Patient Protection and Affordable Care Act of 2010. The complexity is a major issue, but just as much a concern are the tens of billions of dollars spent by government and private entities to set up this new structure. This is money that belongs in the hands of private citizens, not in the hands of government and medical bureaucrats.

CHAPTER 9
AS THE PPACA
CRUMBLES

S ince its passage (some would say, imposition), the PPACA has been crumbling a piece at a time. This is a partial list of provisions that have fallen aside, or assumptions failed to be met…so far.

The PPACA requires every state to offer health insurance to children under 19 without any pre-existing clause. The insurance must be guarantee issue. This means the parents or guardians of a child who has many chronic health conditions could wait to buy insurance until a need arises. As a result, health insurance companies have quit writing coverage for child-only policies. This is an example of a lack of understanding of how health insurance actually works – maybe a nice try, but it has totally failed.

The PPACA removed all caps on lifetime claims, and eliminates annual caps. In the past, limited and affordable health plans could cap annual payments at $50,000, $100,000 or some other amount. The typical standard health insurance policy had a lifetime cap on claims of $3 million or maybe $5 million. Almost no one exceeds these amounts. Yet, by requiring all insurance policies to offer limitless claims, millions suddenly faced losing their limited coverage policies. As a result, the federal government has had to issue more than 1,800 waivers to employers, unions, and even government entities. Democratic Minority Leader Nancy Pelosi said these waivers helped small employers, even though McDonalds, Wal-Mart, the Service Employee International Union, and other mega-organizations have won waivers. The waivers simply show how ill-conceived was this portion of the PPACA.

Another provision, called the CLASS Act (Title 32) required employers to start withholding money from paychecks beginning in 2011 for long term care coverage– unless the employee opted out. The money would go to fund a new federal government benefit that would pay to help someone receive home health care, or long term care in a professional facility. The only problem is that the PPACA directed that all revenue from the CLASS Act tax be used to pay the cost of the new law, and not a dime would go to pay future benefits. The projected tax take was $74 billion over five years. Just recently, the Secretary shut down the program because advisors proved it is not economically feasible.

The PPACA established the Pooled Coverage Insurance Plan (PCIP) to help high risk individuals afford health insurance coverage. It allocated $5 billion in tax dollars the first year, and predicted that by December 2010, 375,000 individuals would enroll. As of July 2011, 32,400 have enrolled. Did Congress overestimate the need or simply stretch the truth just to get a new federal program launched?

Small business, said Congress, would get a hugely popular benefit. The PPACA provides $2 billion to fund tax credits for small business to help pay the insurance premiums of their employees. By June 2011, the federal government projected $435 million will be paid into this program, not $2 billion. Perhaps Congress forgot that in order to benefit from a tax credit, a business had to be profitable. Many small businesses struggle to earn profits, and then they are usually marginal. And most small business operators are notoriously independent and resist government programs, not signing up for them.

The PPACA required employers, starting in 2011, to report on employee's W-2s the total dollars the employer paid for their health care insurance. Soon after passage, the IRS issued a notice that this would not begin in 2011, since they could not figure out how to implement it. The law remains on the books but is not yet enforced.

In November, reports emerged that the Department of Health and Human Services had missed 17 out of 30 statutory requirements. These related to mandatory issuance of rules and regulations, having programs in place, and commissions established. Imagine if you missed buying your license tabs, paying your property taxes, or failing to file income taxes 17 out of 30 times. You would end up in prison, but the Secretary receives nary a hand slap.

The PPACA required all businesses to issue

IRS Form 1099s for every vendor with which they did $600 or more business a year. In the past, this only applied to direct payments that could be classified as income, but not for durable products, supplies, fuel, and so forth. Rosen's Diversified, a food products company in Fairmont, Minnesota, estimated it would go from 1,800 1099s a year under the old law, to 18,000 or more under the new law. To comply with the new law meant Rosen's would have spent the equivalent of 3.5 man-years in wasted salary and benefits. Congress heard the national outcry and rescinded this stupid PPACA provision in 2011.

The PPACA instituted a new tax on July 1, 2010, that required tanning salons to collect a 10 percent tax to help offset the cost of the new health care law. Congress predicted that 25,000 salons would collect $150 million during 2010. Instead, the salons paid in about $54.4 million, and only 10,000 filed the return. The Treasury Department Inspector General for Tax Administration blames IRS "inefficiencies." The IRS is, of course, a branch of the same government that intends to manage your health care. Either the PPACA has caused 15,000 salons to shut down, or turned thousands of entrepreneurs into tax cheats.

MARXISM

The PPACA is political and economic Marxism. It is anti-patient, anti-doctor, anti-elderly, anti-child, and un-American.

Americans should understand how government unions operate. Even private union members know the threat to their future from the power of public unions. Liberals, however, set a goal to eventually turn all health care workers into government union employees.

There are many decent, hardworking government union employees and I respect them. But the structure under which they operate is corrupt and desperately needs reform. We need to privatize as many government run programs as possible.

Government employees were permitted to unionize under President John F. Kennedy. USA Today states that federal government union employees earn between 20 and 40 percent more salary and benefits than their private sector counter-parts. How did this come about?

Generally, every two years government unions negotiate their new salary and benefit package. Union leadership tries to negotiate more pay, less work, more benefits and earlier retirements with paid benefits for their union members. These demands are made regardless of the amount of taxpayer funding available for a particular government program.

I have observed firsthand, as a negotiator for government union contracts for more than six years, how the leaders of state and federal government unions seem at times to deliberately want to bankrupt publicly-supported institutions. The result is that every two years union bosses can show up telling state and federal legislators, "We're broke! We need more money!"

Therefore, no matter how many tax dollars elected officials spend on government programs, it is never enough. They are always short of money and going broke.

The number one employer in the State of Minnesota is the State of Minnesota. The number two employer in Minnesota is the Federal government. This means that those of us who don't work for the government have to work twice as hard to pay for multiple socialistic programs, most of which have a huge amount of waste, fraud, and abuse. And now, add the PPACA to the list.

In addition to this, government union leadership resists changes common to private employers. Union bosses fear that efficiency would result in fewer government union employees. For example, in public education the leadership of the NEA teacher's union supports educational techniques and programs that are inefficient and require an increasing number of government union employees. The unions, for example, want to reduce the teacher's workload to four class periods a day. This means school districts would have to hire more teachers and it means the unions collect more dues.

In general, the union leadership also discouragess audits of government programs that expose waste, fraud, and abuse. The unions can count on some in the media to cover for them.

The Democratic Party (DFL in Minnesota) is the primary recipient of union contributions. The Democrats are often blind proponents of government programs, regardless of the poor results, and generally refuse meaningful reform to change them. In fact, many Democrats and their party leadership support new and expanded government programs with ever more union employees, which in turn creates an increasing stream of political contributions from union dues and members.

Consider so-called welfare programs: When President Obama took office, one of the first things he and the Democrat-controlled congress did was to roll back the requirements to qualify for welfare benefits. This, in turn, leads to more people who are dependent on welfare for their existence, which creates more demand for welfare services, which requires additional government union employees to handle the case loads, who will be forced to join the union and pay union dues, some of which will wind up in the pockets of the liberal Democrats that passed the laws.

ECONOMIC EVIL?

The pillars of the capitalist system, profit and competition, coupled with the rule of law and the possible fear of bankruptcy, produces competitive prices, excellence in services and products, along with increased prosperity for the general population. This is not evil as some liberals imply.

Economic Marxism and socialism, which eliminate the pillars of the capitalistic system, replaces them with substandard and expensive services and products, together with billions of dollars in waste, fraud and abuse: **This is evil**.

WHAT ABOUT OBAMACARE?

Democrats know that when the government runs health care in other nations the record is clear: It always produces rationing and reduces the quality of health care for ill patients. By their actions it appears that the Democrats don't seem to care. Why? If they can eventually turn millions of health care workers into government union employees who will then pay union dues, this will lead to huge political contributions made to Democratic candidates. Whether implicit or explicit, this is the liberal's ultimate goal. Money in politics generates ongoing political power.

If you have your doubts, consider the abortion industry. Many Democrats want to spend tax dollars to fully fund abortions. Furthermore, they want government licensing boards to mandate that medical professionals must perform abortions. Should Democrats be successful in this scheme, it will create many more abortion-related employees, who, subsidized by tax dollars, will contibute more money to the Democratic Party as a result of the shedding of the blood of innocent children.

AS WENT THE MARXIST IDEA, SO GOES THE LIBERAL IDEA

By now I think you get the picture. Liberal Democrats, are willing to bankrupt the United States and destroy the dollar to gain political power. Think of it as a wealthy family. Whoever

ZERO-INTEREST DEFERRED HOME IMPROVEMENT LOANS AVAILABLE IMMEDIATELY TO QUALIFYING HOMEOWNERS

Community Development Block Grant funding is available to assist eligible Coon Rapids property owners fix up their homes.

Eligible households include those at or below 80 percent of area median income. For a household of four in 2012, this income is $65,000. Eligible properties under this program include single- and two-family houses and interior work on townhouses and other common interest community properties. The program focuses on basic home improvements that affect the safety and livability of a structure. Assistance throughout your project, including help developing a written scope of work, is provided by the program administrator.

Funds are made available immediately to qualified applicants on a first-come, first-serve basis. If you feel you could benefit from this program, contact the North Metro Office of the HousingResource Center™ at 651-486-7401 to learn more about this program.

In addition to voting for national, state, and loc
on two constitutional amendments. The first ame
all voters present a valid photo identification to
will ask whether marriage in Minnesota be legall
A YES vote will mean you are in favor of the am
counted as against the amendment.

If you have any questions please contact the Cle
6459.

Getting Ready for Snow...

Winter is just around the corner, and the Ci
of Coon Rapids asks all residents to be aware
some important information that can help us all g
through winter.

Garbage Cart Placement - City guidelines for

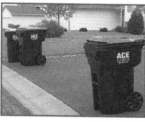

sweeping and plowing
are "curb to curb."
That means, we could
use your help when it
comes to garbage cart
placement, in order the
get the streets as clean
as possible. Please place your cart two feet behind
the curb, with at least three feet in between your
carts. This helps our snow plow drivers plow the
streets thoroughly and clean the streets from
"curb to curb." If the carts are placed in the stree
the plows have to go around them which leaves
that portion of the street incomplete. If you have
~tions on cart placement please call 763-767-

inherits the bulk of the money keeps the power. Control of government equals control of trillions of dollars of inheritance (your tax dollars).

Liberals, despite whether they may be well-meaning, have become brainwashed disciples of a Marxist philosophy that will ultimately reduce us to servitude to the system. As for our health care, it will be in the hands of our rulers and lords. The PPACA will bankrupt this country.

Please, for the sake of your children and grandchildren, become involved at every level and stop the Marxist socialist takeover of our health care system.

Remember the words of Edmund Burke: "The only thing necessary for evil to succeed is for good men to do nothing."

Congress must repeal the PPACA and replace it with true private sector health care reforms that expand patient access to health care and frees the doctor to be a medical professional again. If you love this country, regardless of your political party preference, please contact your state and federally elected representatives and firmly and respectfully voice your opinions on this extremely important health care issue.

You can contact your Representative and Senators by calling the main switchboard at 202-224-3121.

A CALL TO ACTION

Health care deals with the crucible of the human life cycle: birth, sickness, disease, pain and suffering, and finally, death. No book about health care would be complete without addressing the origin of that human dilemma.

There are only three world views on the origin of the human life cycle and all three views are religious. Most people believe in one or a combination of these three world views. Political philosophies of governments are founded on these views or draw significantly from them.

The first world view is that sickness, disease, pain and suffering, and death have always been present in this earth and universe and will always be. When you eventually pass away you are simply extinct. There is no discernible eternal existence therefore, "go for the gusto here on earth for tomorrow you die." This view of origins (macro-evolution) is found in the religion of atheism and supports the political philosophies of communism, Nazism, nihilism, and the like. It also supports centralized government planning of the economy and health care.

The second world view is similar to the first yet distinct. It believes that the life cycle of sickness, disease, pain and suffering, and death has always been and will always be in this earth and universe, but at death, depending on your good works or lack thereof you will "reincarnate" back into the earth and universe. When reincarnated, you will most likely exist in a different form, better or worse than your present existence. This world view is found in most eastern religions such as Hinduism, Buddhism, etc. In the past the political system and laws in India drew heavily on this world view.

The third world view is distinctly different from the first two. It states that sickness, disease, pain and suffering, and death are a consequence imposed by the Creator as a result of the disobedience of mankind. (God created human beings and intended that they would be without sickness and death. He looked on Adam and Eve and pronounced them, "Very good.") This view states that at death individuals enter either eternal salvation or damnation – there is no second chance. This world view also states that one day the Creator will return and make a new heaven and earth that is free from sickness, disease, pain and suffering, and death. Individuals receiving salvation will also be given a new physical body free from the curse of death and decay. This world view has a political philosophy that supports freedom and liberty in natural law and is foundational for a Republic, and ill-suited for a mob democracy. It supports checks and balances on the majority subject to the Creator's revealed law, such as the Ten Commandments. Under this political philosophy, freedom of religion is provided for but limited in action by the Creator's law. For example, human sacrifice is illegal, as is fraud, theft, and perjury.

These three world views stand in opposition to each other. Two of them have to be false and only one can be true. One of them brings comfort to human beings facing sickness, disease, pain and suffering, and death. The other two bring little comfort and result in hopelessness.

> *"Choose you this day whom you will serve: but as for me and my house we will serve the Lord!"*
>
> *Joshua 24:15b*

America, there is a political and spiritual battle going on for the heart and soul of the future of the United States. Please, for the sake of your children and grandchildren, participate in this battle for America's future. From an economic and health care perspective, time is running out.

May God Bless America
Glenn Gruenhagen

RESOURCES

Glenn Gruenhagen, like each of us, relies on many sources to guide him in making wise, informed decisions. As a businessman and a legislator, he has his favorite websites from which to gather information to build his knowledge. These are a few of his favorite websites, and he urges you to begin using them, too:

American Association of Physicians and Surgeons
      http://www.aapsonline.org
Cato Institute
      http://www.cato.org
Center for Medicine in the Public Interest
      http://cmpi.org
Citizens' Council for Health Freedom
      http://www.cchfreedom.org
Coalition for Healthcare Redesign
      http://www.cohronline.com
Free Market Health Care
      http://www.freemarkethealthcare.com
Galen Institute
      http://www.galen.org
Hands off My Health Care
      http://handsoffmyhealth.org
Heartland Institute
      http://heartland.org
National Association of Health Underwriters
      http://www.nahu.org
Nat'l Assn of Insurance and Financial Advisors
      http://www.naifa.org
National Center for Policy Analysis
      http://www.ncpa.org

ABOUT
GLENN GRUENHAGEN

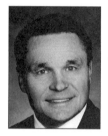

Glenn and Emily Gruenhagen have been married for more than 36 years and live in Glencoe, Minnesota. They have three daughters and five grandchildren.

Glenn grew up on a Minnesota dairy farm. He graduated from Glencoe High School, and attended North Hennepin Junior College, and the University of Minnesota. He holds degrees as a Chartered Financial Consultant (ChFC) and Chartered Life Underwriter (CLU) which he earned from American College, Bryn Mawr, PA.

Shortly after he married Emily, he founded Gruenhagen Insurance and Financial Services. He has worked with hundreds of individuals, couples, families, and small businesses, helping them develop an insurance strategy to protect their assets, and to help them plan for retirement.

Glenn is a veteran of the U.S. Marine Corps and a member of the American Legion. He is a pro-life, pro-family, fiscal conservative. He is a longtime member of the National Rifle Association.

For many years, Glenn has been active in prison ministries, and at Grace Church in Eden Prairie, Minnesota.

Glencoe area voters elected Glenn to the Glencoe Silver Lake Public School Board where he served four terms, a total of 16 years. He is a member of Rotary International.

In 2010, District 25A voters elected Glenn to the Minnesota House of Representatives. In the legislature he serves on four committees: Health and Human Services Reform, Judiciary Policy and Finance, Civil Law, and Public Safety and Crime Prevention Policy and Finance.

To contact Glenn Gruenhagen:

Gruenhagen Insurance and Financial Services
624 E. 13th St., 55336
Phone: 320.864.5903